Norovirus Threat

Navigating the Rise of the Winter Vomiting Bug

Kingsley Freeman

Table of content

<u>Chapter 10: A Call to Action: Empowering Yourself and Your Community</u>

<u>Conclusion</u>

Introduction

In the heart of the winter season, when the air is crisp and the holidays bring families together, a silent threat lurks: norovirus. Often referred to as the "winter vomiting bug" or "stomach flu," norovirus is a highly contagious virus that wreaks havoc on the digestive system, causing vomiting, diarrhea, and stomach cramps. While it's not a new phenomenon, recent data from the Centers for Disease Control and Prevention (CDC) paints a concerning picture: norovirus outbreaks are on the rise in the United States, reaching levels not seen in over a decade.

This book delves into the world of norovirus, exploring its origins, transmission, and the impact it has on individuals and communities. We'll examine the latest trends in norovirus outbreaks, analyze the factors contributing to its spread, and investigate the ongoing search for a vaccine. But this book is more than just a medical report; it's a guide to empower you with the knowledge and tools to protect yourself and your loved ones from this invisible threat.

To understand the magnitude of the norovirus threat, let's look at the numbers. According to the CDC, the first week of December 2023 saw a record-breaking 91 suspected or confirmed norovirus outbreaks, surpassing any previous December reports in over a decade. This surge in cases coincides with a broader trend of increasing seasonal illnesses, as people gather indoors more frequently during the winter months.

The rise of norovirus is part of a larger picture. Many countries are grappling with a surge in seasonal illnesses, including influenza, respiratory syncytial virus (RSV), and even a resurgence of COVID-19. This "quad-demic," as some health experts call it, is putting a strain on healthcare systems and highlighting the importance of prevention and preparedness.
Hope on the Horizon: Vaccines and Research
While there is currently no vaccine specifically for norovirus, researchers are making significant strides in developing one. The pharmaceutical giant Moderna has recently initiated clinical trials for a potential norovirus vaccine, offering a glimmer of hope for future prevention. In the meantime, this book will explore effective strategies for protecting yourself and your loved ones from norovirus and other seasonal illnesses.

This book aims to equip you with the knowledge and tools to navigate the challenges posed by norovirus and other seasonal illnesses. We'll delve into the science behind these viruses, explore effective prevention strategies, and discuss the latest advancements in vaccine development. By understanding the threat and taking proactive steps, we can empower ourselves to stay healthy and protect our communities.
In the following chapters, we will:
 * Explore the science behind norovirus, including its transmission, symptoms, and impact.

* Analyze the latest trends in norovirus outbreaks and the factors contributing to their spread.
* Discuss effective prevention strategies, including handwashing, hygiene practices, and food safety.
* Examine the role of vaccination in preventing other seasonal illnesses.
* Investigate the ongoing research and development of a norovirus vaccine.

By the end of this book, you'll have a comprehensive understanding of norovirus and the tools to protect yourself and your loved ones from this invisible threat. Let's embark on this journey together and empower ourselves to stay healthy in the face of the winter season's challenges.

Chapter 1: The Invisible Enemy: Understanding Norovirus

The air in the pediatrician's office hung thick with the scent of antiseptic and fear. Mrs. Garcia watched her little boy, Leo, curled into a fetal position on the examination table, his face pale and clammy. His small body was wracked with sobs, each one punctuated by a fresh wave of nausea. Dr. Evans, his face etched with concern, gently pressed on Leo's abdomen. "Tell me, Mrs. Garcia," he said, his voice soothing, "when did this all start?"

Mrs. Garcia, her own eyes brimming with worry, recounted the events of the past 24 hours: the sudden onset of vomiting, the explosive diarrhea, the fever that spiked and then vanishes as quickly as it arrived. "He just wouldn't stop throwing up," she whispered, her voice trembling. "I thought it was just a stomach bug, something he picked up at school."

Dr. Evans nodded, his gaze fixed on Leo. "It certainly sounds like it could be," he said, his voice carefully neutral. "Norovirus is going around quite a bit this season."

The word hung in the air, heavy and unfamiliar. Norovirus. What was it? Mrs. Garcia had heard whispers of it at the school drop-off line, a hushed conversation between two other mothers about a particularly virulent strain that had swept through the kindergarten class. But she hadn't given it much thought. Now, faced with her own child's suffering, the word took on a terrifying new meaning.

Leaving the doctor's office, Mrs. Garcia clutched Leo close, his small body still trembling. The afternoon sun, a pale imitation of its usual brilliance, cast long shadows across the sidewalk. As she walked, she tried to piece together the puzzle of this invisible enemy. What exactly was norovirus? How had it invaded her son's life so suddenly and violently?

Norovirus, she learned later that evening, is a highly contagious virus that attacks the lining of the stomach and intestines. It's a microscopic beast, a tiny, resilient particle that can cause a whirlwind of unpleasant symptoms. Unlike the flu, which is caused by a different type of virus, norovirus doesn't target the respiratory system. Instead, it wreaks havoc on the digestive tract, leading to a cascade of unpleasant effects.

The virus spreads with astonishing ease. It can be transmitted through contaminated food or water, but also through close contact with infected individuals. Tiny particles of the virus can linger on surfaces, waiting to be transferred to unsuspecting hands. A handshake, a shared utensil, even a doorknob can become a vector for this insidious disease.

The symptoms of norovirus are as dramatic as they are unpleasant. Sudden and explosive vomiting is often the first sign, followed closely by watery diarrhea. Abdominal cramps can be excruciating, and many people experience nausea, headache, and even fever. The illness typically lasts for one to three days, but the weakness and fatigue can linger for much longer.

Mrs. Garcia, as she watched Leo sleep fitfully that night, couldn't help but wonder how her son had contracted the virus. Had he eaten something contaminated at school? Had he touched a contaminated surface and then unknowingly transferred the virus to his mouth? The questions swirled in her mind, each unanswered question adding to her anxiety.

Norovirus, she realized, was a silent and insidious enemy, a microscopic invader that could strike at any moment, disrupting lives and leaving a trail of misery in its wake. It was a stark reminder of the fragility of health and the constant vigilance required to protect ourselves and our loved ones from the invisible threats that surround us.

The following morning, as Leo's fever subsided and the vomiting finally ceased, Mrs. Garcia began to understand the true nature of the enemy she faced. Norovirus, she realized, was not just a "stomach bug," a minor inconvenience to be shrugged off. It was a formidable opponent, a microscopic adversary that could bring even the strongest among us to our knees.

The virus, she learned, is incredibly resilient. It can survive harsh conditions, remaining viable on surfaces for extended periods. Even after a thorough cleaning, traces of the virus can linger, waiting for the next unsuspecting victim. This resilience made it incredibly difficult to contain outbreaks, especially in crowded settings such as schools, daycare centers, and hospitals.

One of the most concerning aspects of norovirus is its remarkable ability to spread rapidly through populations. A single infected individual can easily contaminate food, water, and surfaces, leading to a chain reaction of infections. Outbreaks can occur in a matter of hours, sweeping through households, schools, and even entire communities.

The impact of a norovirus outbreak can be significant. Schools may be forced to close temporarily, businesses may experience disruptions, and healthcare systems can become overwhelmed. The economic and social costs of these outbreaks can be substantial, highlighting the importance of prevention and control measures.

As Mrs. Garcia watched Leo cautiously sip some clear fluids, she vowed to learn everything she could about this invisible enemy. She knew that protecting her family from norovirus would require vigilance, meticulous hygiene practices, and a thorough understanding of how this insidious virus spread.

The experience had been a wake-up call. The invisible world of viruses, once a distant concern, had suddenly become a very real and present danger. Norovirus, she realized, was not just a medical term in a textbook; it was a force to be reckoned with, a silent threat that could disrupt lives and challenge even the most robust defenses.

Chapter 2: The Norovirus Outbreak: A Silent Tsunami

The news of the outbreak hit Sarah like a rogue wave. One minute she was bustling around the kitchen, preparing lunch for her two young children, the next she was staring at the school's emergency notification on her phone. "Norovirus outbreak in Mrs. Peterson's second-grade class," the message read. "Please keep your child home if they exhibit any symptoms."

A wave of dread washed over her. Norovirus. The word, once a distant echo in the back of her mind, now loomed large, a menacing specter threatening to disrupt her family's routine. Images of her children, pale and listless, curled up in bed, flashed through her mind. The thought of their tiny bodies ravaged by nausea and diarrhea filled her with a primal fear.

She glanced at her children, who were engrossed in a playful wrestling match on the living room floor. Their laughter, once a source of joy, now seemed fragile, easily shattered by the invisible threat lurking just beyond their reach. Sarah's gaze fell on the doorknobs, the countertops, the toys scattered across the floor — potential breeding grounds for the insidious virus.

The school was quick to act. Within hours, the news of the outbreak had spread through the parent grapevine, a silent, yet palpable wave of anxiety rippling through the community. Playdates were canceled, birthday parties postponed, and social gatherings were met with a cautious hesitation. The air was thick with worry, a collective unease hanging heavy over the neighborhood. Sarah spent the next few days on high alert. She washed her hands obsessively, disinfecting every surface within reach. She monitored her children closely, watching for any signs of illness: a sudden pallor, a hint of nausea, a rumbling stomach. The fear, once a distant tremor, had now escalated into a full-blown panic.

The outbreak, however, was relentless. It spread through the school like wildfire, leaping from classroom to classroom, leaving a trail of sick children in its wake. The school nurse's office became a makeshift triage center, overwhelmed with vomiting children and anxious parents. The atmosphere in the school hallways was a strange mix of fear and resignation, a collective sigh of surrender to the invisible enemy.The impact of the outbreak extended beyond the school walls. Local businesses, particularly restaurants and cafes, experienced a sharp decline in foot traffic as parents kept their children home and avoided public spaces. The community, once vibrant and bustling, now wore a mask of caution, each interaction tinged with a subtle undercurrent of fear.

Sarah, like many other parents, found herself caught in a whirlwind of anxiety and uncertainty. She juggled the demands of work with the constant vigilance required to protect her children. Sleep eluded her, replaced by a constant state of hyper-awareness, her senses on high alert for any sign of illness.

The outbreak, she realized, was more than just a nuisance. It was a disruptive force, a silent tsunami that had swept through her community, leaving a trail of disruption and anxiety in its wake. The invisible enemy, once a distant threat, had now become a very real and present danger, a constant reminder of the fragility of health and the importance of preparedness.

As the days passed, the outbreak began to subside, the initial wave of panic gradually giving way to a sense of weary relief. But the experience had left an indelible mark on Sarah and her community. The invisible enemy, once a distant threat, had now become a very real and present danger, a constant reminder of the fragility of health and the importance of preparedness.

Chapter 3: The "Quad-demic" and Beyond: A Winter of Illnesses

The air in the emergency room felt thick with the scent of antiseptic and fear. Dr. Anya Sharma, her face etched with exhaustion, navigated the maze of beds, each one occupied by a patient battling a different facet of the winter illness surge. A child coughed raucously in one bed, their tiny chest heaving with each labored breath. In the next, an elderly woman lay shivering, her skin clammy and pale, battling a severe case of influenza.

This was the new reality, Dr. Sharma thought, a grim reflection of the winter of illnesses that had descended upon the city. Norovirus, once a distant threat, had joined forces with other formidable foes: influenza, respiratory syncytial virus (RSV), and the ever-present COVID-19. The result was a perfect storm, a confluence of illnesses that was overwhelming hospitals and straining healthcare systems to their limits.

The hallways, once bustling with activity, now resembled a war zone. Nurses rushed from room to room, their faces masked, their eyes filled with a weary determination. The air crackled with the urgency of the situation, each cough, each labored breath a stark reminder of the invisible enemies that were besieging the city.

Dr. Sharma moved from patient to patient, her hands a blur of motion as she checked vitals, administered medications, and offered words of comfort. Each patient was a unique story, a testament to the resilience of the human spirit in the face of adversity. But the sheer volume of patients was overwhelming, pushing the hospital staff to their physical and emotional limits.

The situation was mirrored across the country, and indeed, around the globe. Hospitals in major cities were overflowing, beds were scarce, and staff were stretched thin. The winter of illnesses was not just a local phenomenon; it was a global crisis, a stark reminder of the interconnectedness of the human race and the vulnerability of our health systems.In Europe, the situation was particularly dire. Countries across the continent were grappling with a surge in influenza cases, with some regions reporting record-breaking numbers. The NHS in England, already under immense strain, was struggling to cope with the influx of patients. Hospitals were operating at overcapacity, with ambulances often forced to queue outside, unable to offload patients due to a lack of available beds.

In Asia, the resurgence of COVID-19, fueled by new variants, was adding further strain to already overburdened healthcare systems. In some countries, the healthcare infrastructure was simply unable to cope with the surge in demand, leading to widespread shortages of beds, ventilators, and essential medical supplies.

The winter of illnesses was not just a medical crisis; it was a social and economic crisis as well. Schools were forced to close, businesses were disrupted, and travel plans were thrown into disarray. The fear and uncertainty that had gripped communities during the early days of the pandemic returned with a vengeance, casting a long shadow over daily life.

Dr. Sharma, as she navigated the chaos of the emergency room, couldn't help but reflect on the fragility of human health and the interconnectedness of the world. The winter of illnesses was a stark reminder that the invisible enemies that surround us can quickly overwhelm even the most robust healthcare systems. It was a call to action, a plea for greater preparedness, and a reminder of the importance of global cooperation in the face of shared threats.

Chapter 4: The Enemy Within: How Norovirus Spreads

The lunchroom at Elmwood Elementary buzzed with the usual cacophony of sounds: the clatter of trays, the excited chatter of children, the low hum of adult voices. Little Lily, oblivious to the invisible threat lurking amidst the lunchtime chaos, happily devoured her peanut butter and jelly sandwich, occasionally sharing bites with her best friend, Emily.

Across the table, Emily, already feeling a tickle in her throat, unknowingly touched her face, then reached for the shared bag of apple slices. The virus, a microscopic hitchhiker, clung tenaciously to her fingers, ready to embark on its next journey.

This seemingly innocuous exchange, a moment of childhood camaraderie, would soon have far-reaching consequences. As Emily unknowingly ingested the virus, the chain of transmission had begun.

Norovirus, a cunning adversary, exploits the most mundane of human interactions. It hitches a ride on contaminated hands, spreads through droplets expelled during coughing or sneezing, and lurks within contaminated food and water. Its pathways are diverse and often invisible, making it a formidable opponent to contain.

The virus can survive for extended periods on surfaces, clinging tenaciously to doorknobs, countertops, and even the plastic surfaces of toys. A child, playing innocently with a contaminated toy, can easily transfer the virus to their hands and then to their mouth, unwittingly setting off a new wave of infections.

Food, a source of sustenance, can also become a vehicle for the virus. Contaminated shellfish, fruits, and vegetables can harbor the virus, waiting to unleash its insidious effects upon unsuspecting consumers. Outbreaks linked to contaminated food are not uncommon, often occurring in restaurants, schools, and other settings where food is prepared and served.

But norovirus is not merely a passive passenger; it is an active participant in its own dissemination. The virus, expelled from the body through vomit and diarrhea, can contaminate surrounding surfaces and even the air. These microscopic particles, laden with infectious material, can travel short distances, infecting others in close proximity.

This phenomenon, known as "respiratory droplet transmission," plays a significant role in the rapid spread of norovirus in crowded settings such as schools, daycare centers, and cruise ships. The confined spaces, coupled with the high density of people, create an ideal environment for the virus to thrive and multiply.

The virus, a master of disguise, can also be transmitted through seemingly innocuous means. A shared water bottle, a forgotten toothbrush, even a handshake can become a conduit for infection. The virus, ever vigilant, seeks out new hosts, exploiting every opportunity to expand its reach.

The invisible pathways of norovirus transmission are a constant reminder of the fragility of human health and the importance of vigilance. From contaminated surfaces to shared utensils, from respiratory droplets to contaminated food, the virus lurks everywhere, waiting for the next unsuspecting victim.

Understanding these pathways is crucial in the fight against norovirus. By recognizing the diverse and often invisible ways in which the virus spreads, we can implement effective prevention strategies, minimizing its impact and protecting ourselves and our communities.

Chapter 5: Symptoms Revealed: Recognizing the Norovirus Invasion

The first sign was a rumbling in her stomach, a low growl that quickly escalated into a full-blown crescendo. Lily, curled up on the living room rug, clutching her stuffed panda, felt a wave of nausea wash over her. She squeezed her eyes shut, her breath catching in her throat.

Her mother, sensing her distress, rushed to her side. "Lily, sweetheart, what's wrong?" she asked, her voice laced with concern.

Lily, unable to speak, simply pointed towards the bathroom, her face pale and drawn. As she stumbled towards the bathroom, a wave of dizziness washed over her, and she collapsed onto the cold tiles, her stomach heaving.

The next few hours were a blur of vomiting, diarrhea, and debilitating cramps. Lily, weak and listless, lay huddled in her bed, her body wracked with chills. Her mother, a constant presence by her side, watched helplessly as the virus, a relentless adversary, took its toll.

Norovirus, once an invisible threat, had now manifested itself in a terrifyingly tangible way. The initial symptoms, often sudden and explosive, could be alarming. Vomiting, a forceful and unrelenting expulsion of stomach contents, was a hallmark of the infection. This was often accompanied by watery diarrhea, which could be frequent and profuse.

Abdominal cramps, a constant, gnawing pain, added to the misery. The muscles of the abdomen would contract and spasm, each wave of pain leaving Lily gasping for breath.

But the physical symptoms were only part of the story. Norovirus, like a skilled puppeteer, could also manipulate the senses, creating a symphony of unpleasant sensations. Nausea, a persistent feeling of queasiness, lingered in the background, a constant reminder of the virus's presence.

Fatigue, a debilitating weakness, settled over the body, leaving the victim feeling drained and listless. Even the simplest of tasks, such as getting out of bed or walking to the bathroom, seemed like monumental efforts.In some cases, the virus could also cause fever, headache, and muscle aches, adding another layer of discomfort to the already debilitating symptoms. The illness, though typically short-lived, could leave its victims feeling weak and exhausted for days, a lingering reminder of the virus's potent effects.

As Lily lay in bed, her body weakened by the virus, she felt a sense of isolation, a feeling of being cut off from the world. The vibrant colors of the outside world seemed muted, replaced by a hazy gray. The sounds of laughter and play, once a source of joy, now seemed distant and unreal.

The virus, it seemed, had not only attacked her body but also her spirit, leaving her feeling vulnerable and helpless. But even in the midst of her illness, a flicker of hope remained. The virus, though powerful, was not invincible. With rest, hydration, and supportive care, she would recover, stronger and more resilient than before.

The experience, however, had left an indelible mark. The invisible enemy, once a distant threat, had now become a terrifying reality, a stark reminder of the vulnerability of the human body and the importance of taking care of oneself.

Chapter 6: Fortified Defense: Protecting Yourself from Norovirus

The memory of her son's illness still lingered, a haunting reminder of the invisible enemy that had invaded their lives. Sarah, determined to protect her family from future outbreaks, embarked on a mission to fortify their defenses against norovirus.

The first line of defense, she knew, was a simple yet crucial one: handwashing. She transformed handwashing into a ritual, a sacred practice that was observed with meticulous attention to detail.

"Hands, hands, hands," she would chant, her voice a gentle mantra as she guided her children through the proper handwashing technique. "Lather up for at least 20 seconds, scrubbing between your fingers, under your nails, and around your wrists."

She stocked up on hand sanitizer, placing bottles strategically throughout the house – by the front door, in the kitchen, and even in the children's backpacks. The act of sanitizing hands became a reflexive action, a subconscious response to the ever-present threat of the virus.

Disinfecting surfaces became another crucial component of their defense strategy. Sarah meticulously cleaned and disinfected all high-touch surfaces throughout the house, from doorknobs and light switches to countertops and toys.

She even implemented a "shoe-off" policy at the front door, a small but significant step in preventing the virus from being tracked into the house on the soles of shoes. Food safety became a paramount concern. Fruits and vegetables were washed thoroughly before consumption, and meat and poultry were cooked to the proper temperature. Leftovers were stored promptly in the refrigerator, minimizing the risk of bacterial growth.

Sarah also implemented a strict "no sharing" policy regarding food and drinks. Each child had their own utensils, plates, and cups, minimizing the risk of cross-contamination.

These measures, though seemingly small, were a testament to Sarah's determination to protect her family. She had transformed her home into a fortress, a sanctuary shielded from the invisible threat of norovirus.

The experience had taught her a valuable lesson: the fight against norovirus was a constant, vigilant struggle, a never-ending effort to outsmart an invisible enemy. By implementing these simple yet effective measures, she had empowered herself and her family to take control of their health and minimize their risk of infection.

The memory of her son's illness, though painful, had served as a powerful motivator, driving her to take proactive steps to protect her loved ones. She had learned that even the smallest of actions, when taken collectively, could make a significant difference in the fight against this insidious disease.

Chapter 7: Navigating Outbreaks: Staying Safe in Public Spaces

The news of the outbreak at Sunnyside Preschool sent a wave of panic through the neighborhood. Children, who had been playing carefree in the park just hours before, were now confined to their homes, their laughter replaced by the muffled sounds of cartoons and the occasional sniffle.

Sarah, like many other parents, found herself navigating a new set of challenges. How could she keep her children safe while still maintaining a semblance of normalcy in their lives?

The playground, once a haven of joy and social interaction, now seemed like a minefield, a potential breeding ground for infection. Playdates, once eagerly anticipated, were met with a cautious hesitation. The fear of the invisible enemy, lurking in every shared toy, every lingering cough, cast a long shadow over their social interactions.

Sarah began to approach public spaces with a newfound caution. She scrutinized surfaces before allowing her children to touch them, wiping down stroller handles and playground equipment with disinfectant wipes. She encouraged her children to wash their hands frequently, especially after playing in public spaces.

The school, in an effort to contain the outbreak, implemented strict hygiene protocols. Hand sanitizer dispensers were placed strategically throughout the school, and regular hand washing breaks were incorporated into the daily schedule. The school cafeteria, once a bustling hub of activity, now wore a mask of caution, with tables spaced further apart and food served in individual containers.

Despite these measures, the outbreak continued to spread, a relentless tide that threatened to overwhelm the school. The school administration, faced with a growing number of sick children, made the difficult decision to temporarily close the school, a move that sent ripples of anxiety through the community.

The closure of the school, however, presented a new set of challenges. With both parents working, finding childcare during the unexpected closure was a logistical nightmare. Sarah, like many other parents, found herself scrambling to make arrangements, juggling work responsibilities with the demands of childcare.

The outbreak, she realized, was not just a medical crisis; it was a social and economic crisis as well. It disrupted routines, strained relationships, and added a layer of stress to an already demanding lifestyle.But amidst the chaos, there were also glimmers of hope. The community, faced with a shared threat, rallied together. Neighbors offered to help with childcare, parents shared resources, and a sense of solidarity emerged, a testament to the resilience of the human spirit in the face of adversity.

Chapter 8: The Search for a Solution: The Quest for a Norovirus Vaccine

Dr. Eleanor Vance, a virologist at a leading research institution, stared intently at the electron micrograph, the image of the norovirus magnified thousands of times. The virus, a tiny, resilient particle, seemed to mock her from the screen, a constant reminder of the challenges that lay ahead.

Years of research had yielded little progress in the development of a norovirus vaccine. The virus, with its remarkable ability to mutate and evade the immune response, proved to be a formidable opponent.

"It's like trying to hit a moving target," Dr. Vance muttered to herself, frustration creeping into her voice. "The virus is constantly changing, adapting, evolving."

Despite the challenges, the quest for a norovirus vaccine continued with renewed vigor. Scientists, driven by a sense of urgency and a deep-seated desire to protect public health, were exploring new avenues of research.

One promising approach involved developing vaccines that target the conserved regions of the virus, the parts of the viral structure that remain relatively unchanged despite mutations. By focusing on these conserved regions, researchers hoped to create vaccines that would provide broad protection against a wide range of norovirus strains.

Another promising avenue of research involved the use of novel vaccine technologies, such as mRNA vaccines. These innovative vaccines, which have shown remarkable success in the fight against COVID-19, could potentially be adapted to target norovirus.

The road ahead, however, was fraught with challenges. The development of a safe and effective vaccine would require years of rigorous research, extensive clinical trials, and significant investment in scientific research.

But Dr. Vance, despite the challenges, remained optimistic. "We will find a way," she declared, her voice filled with determination. "We will not give up until we have conquered this elusive enemy."

The quest for a norovirus vaccine was a testament to the resilience of the human spirit, a relentless pursuit of knowledge in the face of adversity. It was a reminder that even the most formidable challenges could be overcome through perseverance, innovation, and a commitment to improving human health.

The future of norovirus prevention, Dr. Vance believed in continued research, collaborative efforts, and an unwavering commitment to scientific discovery. The journey may be long and arduous, but the potential rewards a world free from the threat of norovirus were well worth the effort

Chapter 9: Beyond Norovirus: The Importance of Vaccination

Dr. Emily Carter, a pediatrician at a bustling children's clinic, watched as a stream of parents brought their children in for their routine vaccinations. The clinic, a vibrant hub of childhood development, was a testament to the power of preventive medicine.

"It's amazing," she thought to herself, watching a young mother cradle her infant son while the nurse administered a series of vaccinations. "These tiny needles are protecting these children from a host of serious illnesses."

Vaccinations, Dr. Carter knew, were a cornerstone of modern medicine, a powerful tool in the fight against infectious diseases. They had eradicated diseases that once ravaged communities, such as smallpox and polio, and had significantly reduced the burden of other serious illnesses, such as measles, mumps, and rubella.

"Every vaccination," she often told parents, "is a small victory in the battle against disease."

The benefits of vaccination extended beyond individual health. By increasing herd immunity, vaccinations protect not only the vaccinated individuals but also those who are unable to be vaccinated, such as infants, immunocompromised individuals, and pregnant women.

Dr. Carter often emphasized the importance of vaccinating children according to the recommended schedule. This, she explained, would provide them with the best possible protection against a range of childhood diseases, including measles, mumps, rubella, polio, diphtheria, tetanus, pertussis, and chickenpox.

But the benefits of vaccination extended beyond childhood. Adults too, needed to stay up-to-date on their vaccinations. The flu vaccine, for example, was crucial in preventing severe illness, hospitalization, and even death, particularly among the elderly and those with underlying health conditions.

The COVID-19 pandemic had underscored the critical importance of vaccination in protecting public health. The rapid development and deployment of COVID-19 vaccines had been a remarkable achievement, a testament to the power of scientific innovation and global collaboration.

Dr. Carter, as she administered vaccines to her young patients, felt a sense of pride and responsibility. She was not just a doctor; she was a guardian, a protector, a frontline soldier in the battle against disease.

The fight against infectious diseases, she knew, was a continuous and evolving one. New vaccines were constantly being developed, and existing vaccines were continually being refined and improved.

The future of public health, she believed, depended on continued investment in vaccination research, widespread access to vaccines, and a commitment to public health education. By working together, she believed, we could create a healthier future for generations to come.

As she watched the children leave her clinic, their faces beaming with health and vitality, Dr. Carter felt a sense of satisfaction. She knew that each vaccination was a small but significant step towards a healthier future, a future where the specter of infectious diseases would be a distant memory.

Chapter 10: A Call to Action: Empowering Yourself and Your Community

The memory of the norovirus outbreak, the lingering fear of the "quad-demic," and the ongoing struggle against other infectious diseases had left an indelible mark on Sarah. It had transformed her from a concerned parent to an advocate for public health.

She began to share her experiences with other parents, organizing community workshops on handwashing, hygiene, and the importance of vaccination. She volunteered at local health clinics, assisting with outreach programs and educating the community about the importance of preventive measures.

She joined local advocacy groups, working alongside other concerned citizens to raise awareness about the importance of public health initiatives. She wrote letters to her elected officials, urging them to increase funding for public health programs, support vaccine research, and improve access to healthcare for all.

Sarah's efforts, though small, were a testament to the power of individual action. She had learned that even the smallest of actions, when taken collectively, could have a significant impact on public health.

The fight against infectious diseases, she realized, was not just the responsibility of healthcare professionals and government officials. It was a collective responsibility, a shared endeavor that required the active participation of every member of the community.

By empowering ourselves with knowledge, taking proactive steps to protect our own health, and advocating for public health policies, we could create a more resilient and healthier future for ourselves and for generations to come.

The journey had been challenging, filled with uncertainties and anxieties. But it had also been a journey of growth, a testament to the resilience of the human spirit. Sarah, once a concerned parent, had emerged as a powerful advocate, a voice for change in her community.

The future, she knew, held both challenges and opportunities. But with vigilance, resilience, and a commitment to collective action, we could navigate the challenges, overcome the obstacles, and build a healthier, more equitable future for all.

The fight against infectious diseases, she realized, was a marathon, not a sprint. It required sustained effort, unwavering commitment, and a deep-seated belief in the power of collective action. But the rewards, a healthier future for all, were well worth the effort.

The journey had just begun.

Conclusion

The journey through the world of norovirus and the broader landscape of infectious diseases has been a sobering one. We have witnessed the devastating impact of these invisible enemies – the disruption of daily life, the strain on healthcare systems, and the emotional toll on individuals and communities.

From the initial fear and uncertainty surrounding the norovirus outbreak to the collective struggle against a "quad-demic" of winter illnesses, we have seen firsthand the challenges that these invisible threats pose. We have explored the intricate pathways of norovirus transmission, the debilitating symptoms of infection, and the tireless efforts of scientists and healthcare professionals to combat these insidious diseases.

The quest for a norovirus vaccine, a beacon of hope in the face of uncertainty, has underscored the importance of scientific innovation and the relentless pursuit of knowledge. We have also witnessed the power of vaccination in preventing other serious illnesses, a testament to the remarkable achievements of modern medicine.

But this book is not merely a chronicle of disease; it is a call to action. It is a call to empower ourselves and our communities to take proactive steps in the face of these invisible threats.

 * Individual Responsibility: We must prioritize personal hygiene, practicing diligent hand washing and disinfecting frequently touched surfaces. We must be

mindful of food safety practices and avoid sharing food or drinks with others.

* Collective Action: We must support public health initiatives, advocate for increased funding for vaccine research, and ensure equitable access to healthcare for all.

* Community Resilience: We must foster a sense of community, supporting each other during outbreaks and ensuring that vulnerable populations have the resources they need to stay healthy.

The fight against infectious diseases is a continuous and evolving one. It requires vigilance, resilience, and a commitment to collective action. It requires us to be informed, to be proactive, and to be compassionate.

The future holds both challenges and opportunities. We may face new and emerging threats, but we also possess the knowledge, the tools, and the collective will to overcome these challenges.

This book is not an endpoint; it is a starting point. It is a call to action, an invitation to join the fight against infectious diseases, to become part of the solution. By working together, by empowering ourselves and our communities, we can build a healthier, more resilient future for all. The End

www.ingramcontent.com/pod-product-compliance
Lightning Source LLC
Chambersburg PA
CBHW051721250726